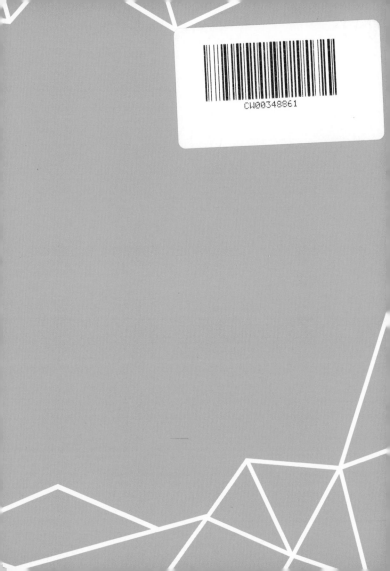

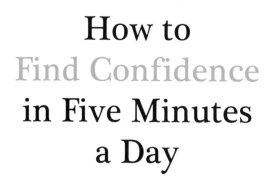

How to Find Confidence in Five Minutes a Day

A Woman's Guide to Self-Love

OLIVIA ROBERTS

HOW TO FIND CONFIDENCE IN FIVE MINUTES A DAY

Text by Caitlin McAllister

An Hachette UK Company
www.hachette.co.uk

Vie Books, an imprint of Summersdale Publishers
Part of Octopus Publishing Group Limited
Carmelite House
50 Victoria Embankment
LONDON
EC4Y 0DZ
UK

www.summersdale.com

Printed and bound in China

ISBN: 978-1-83799-375-8

Substantial discounts on bulk quantities of Summersdale books are available to corporations, professional associations and other organizations. For details contact general enquiries: telephone: +44 (0) 1243 771107 or email: enquiries@summersdale.com.

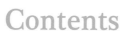

Contents

Introduction

Have you ever been too nervous to raise your hand or share a great idea in front of a crowd? Maybe you listen to your inner critic too much, or perhaps your self-esteem is at an all-time low. If any of these apply to you, you should know two things: you are not the only one feeling this way, and you don't need to feel this way forever.

Self-love is one of life's most important lessons, yet so many of us – especially women – struggle to learn it. There is a clear imbalance between women's and men's confidence levels and in how they feel about themselves. While women regularly show love to their families and friends, they rarely extend the same kindness to themselves. This experience is well documented as an issue facing women in all walks of life.

The thoughts and suggestions in this book provide actionable advice that can be practised every day to help you find your voice, realize your worth and follow your dreams. By the end of the book, you will feel more comfortable in your own skin, have genuine adoration for all the little things that make you "you", and be ready to start confidently working towards your goals.

You are perfectly cast in your life. I can't imagine anyone but you in the role. Go play.

LIN-MANUEL MIRANDA

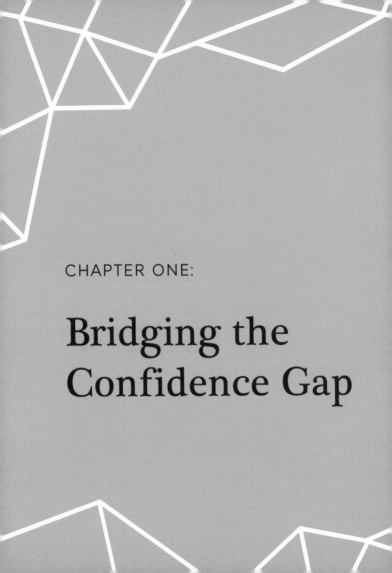

CHAPTER ONE:

Bridging the
Confidence Gap

Not-so-fun fact: men are more likely to self-promote than women are. This is called the "confidence gap", and it's a real thing. In fact, studies have found that at all stages of life, and in multiple career fields and situations, women tend to hang back and avoid putting themselves forward for opportunities, while men feel more comfortable going after what they want.

In this chapter, you will learn simple tips to help you recognize what's holding your confidence back and what you can do to start building it. By taking these first steps, you'll be closer to closing the confidence gap for good.

We all deserve to
live each day as
the best version
of ourselves

Meet your
inner shy girl

In order to find your confidence, the first thing you need to do is identify the obstacles standing in your way — which means it's time to quiz your inner shy girl.

Try carving out some time each day to reflect on your confidence levels — it might be helpful to do this last thing at night before you go to bed. Take a piece of paper and write down a few prompts for yourself, such as: "I tend to feel shyest when..." or "I feel my least confident when...". You can use your experiences from that day to help you.

Once you've done that, you can start writing about when you feel your most confident. Identifying this will make you think about how you can approach the things that drain your confidence and how you can do more of the things that boost it. By practising this every day, you can read back what you've written and see how much your confidence has grown over time.

Find out who you are
and do it on purpose.

DOLLY PARTON

Find your
hidden confidence

Feeling like you lack confidence usually means it is hiding somewhere within you. For example, perhaps you feel unconfident sharing your ideas in a meeting, but you do feel confident that you are very good at your job overall. Similarly, you might feel unconfident planning work projects, but when it comes to travelling abroad solo, you feel your most confident, energized and secure. Lacking confidence in some areas doesn't mean you don't have any, it just means your confidence is hiding somewhere else. By focusing on the things you are confident in, and using the tips inside this book every day, you'll be amazed by the new heights your self-worth will reach.

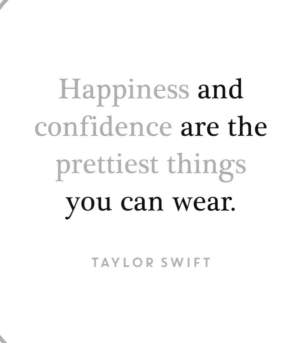

Happiness **and** confidence **are the** prettiest things **you can wear.**

TAYLOR SWIFT

I am worthy of
every magical
thing this world
has to offer

Practise
positive self-talk

Positive self-talk can act as a catalyst for our confidence, and it's why things like affirmations and gratitude work so well. Speaking to yourself with kindness has been proven to have many benefits — not only can it improve your well-being, it can also enhance your performance at work and in your studies.

There is no end to what positive self-talk can do for your confidence, so try practising it every day. If it helps, you could try writing down what you'd like to say and reading it aloud. This could be specific to a situation you feel unconfident in, such as "I'm going to knock this exam out of the park!", or a general statement that could kick-start your confidence, such as "I can totally do this." In time, this will become your mantra.

Get to
know yourself

The journey to acquiring more confidence often leads to us questioning other aspects of our personality. Why do we feel the need to improve our confidence? What is it we most want out of life? Who are we when we strip away the layers? Here are a few things you might want to try, even if only for 5 minutes a day:

- Reflect on your life so far — **What has been good? What has been bad? What did you once believe that you no longer do, and vice versa? Ask yourself these questions while journalling and you are sure to discover new depths to your personality.**

- Try new things — **You never know what you might like until you try it, so if there's anything you have always been curious about, go for it.**

- Practise mindfulness — **Being present in the moment is an excellent skill to develop, and can give you the time and space to really get to know and feel comfortable with yourself. You don't have to become a meditation expert in order to experience mindfulness, either; something as simple as focusing on your breathing for 5 minutes while in the shower or waiting for the kettle to boil can be all you need.**

To love oneself
is the beginning of
a lifelong romance.

OSCAR WILDE

Rate your confidence

Before you dive into your confidence-building journey, rate where you think your confidence is right now on a scale of one to ten. You could choose to rate your general confidence or your specific reason for picking up this book: for example, to improve your confidence in social settings. Consider things like why you feel drawn to improve your confidence at this point in your life, and how the confidence gap may have held you back so far. Make a note of this rating and anything else that might be relevant. After a few weeks or months, once you've developed a confidence routine based on the tips and advice in this book, you can refer back to your rating and see how your confidence has grown.

Eliminate imposter syndrome

Imposter syndrome is the feeling of being an "imposter", or not being qualified to be in the job or position you are in. It's a common feeling that affects many people, even some of the highest achievers.

Imposter syndrome causes us to doubt our intellect, accomplishments and skills, even when there is no reason to. This can lead to feelings of nervousness in our day-to-day life. You might experience negative self-talk that tells you you are "a fraud" or "just lucky" when answering questions correctly.

Imposter syndrome makes us believe we don't deserve to have the position we have, but learning to recognize it in the moment can help us to overcome it. To avoid imposter syndrome creeping in, try repeating the following affirmations to yourself every day:

- "I have as much right to be here as everyone else."
- "I have studied this subject for years. I know what I'm talking about."
- "I am no less capable than anyone else."

LOVE YOURSELF FIRST
AND EVERYTHING
ELSE FALLS INTO LINE.
YOU REALLY HAVE TO
LOVE YOURSELF TO
GET ANYTHING DONE
IN THIS WORLD.

LUCILLE BALL

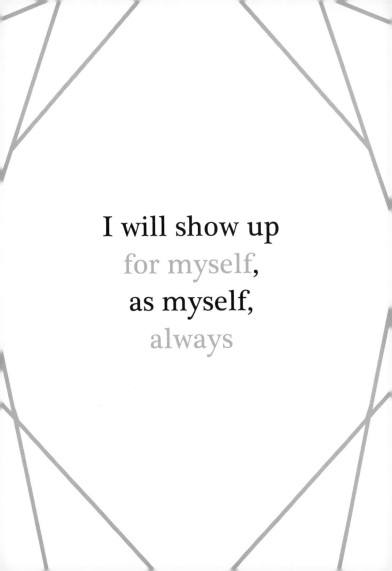

I will show up
for myself,
as myself,
always

Learn to say yes

When we lack confidence, saying yes can sometimes feel like a BIG deal. We may not want to commit to anything outside of our comfort zone, or we could feel uncomfortable saying yes before we know the exact details of what we are agreeing to.

Remember, the things worth doing in life exist on the outskirts of our comfort zone, and to get to those things, sometimes we have to say yes.

Closing the confidence gap means taking all of the amazing experiences life has to offer, so it can help to get used to saying yes at least sometimes. Even if it feels uncomfortable or scary in the moment, it has the potential to bring you a whole lot of happiness further down the line. Try making a conscious effort each day to say yes to the opportunities you would usually shy away from. Whether it's taking on a new work project or accepting an invitation to a party, throwing yourself into something new boosts your confidence by making you realize just how much you're capable of.

Channel "main character energy"

Have you ever felt like the "best friend" character? You know, the one in all the rom-coms who is there to support the main character on all their adventures and basically exists only to help the protagonist move their story along.

Well, it's time to be less of a best friend and more of a main character in your own story. You are just as deserving of a primary storyline, so live every day as the protagonist of your own life — whether that means taking yourself on a date or updating your wardrobe to fit your vision of yourself. You do you!

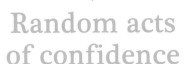

Random acts of confidence

Small acts of confidence scattered throughout your day all add up to something big in the long run, and slowly build your self-belief. For example, if you lack confidence in the gym, set yourself a challenge to ask one of the instructors how to use a new piece of equipment. If you struggle with speaking to new people, try asking your barista, "How are you today?" when buying your morning coffee. Or, if you want to share your ideas more confidently at work, start by sharing low-importance ideas like suggesting a good place to order lunch from.

Just one small act of confidence every day will continually boost your self-belief on an ongoing basis.

The most beautiful thing
you can wear is confidence.

BLAKE LIVELY

Affirmations for focus

Affirmations can be powerful tools to convince your brain of the reality you want to manifest, and you'll find them throughout this book. When our self-belief is lacking and our mental focus is waning on the journey to reach our goals, affirmations have the potential to steady our mindset and boost our confidence. Here are a few that could help you maintain focus if you recite them every day:

- "I'm making amazing progress. Everything I do brings me one step closer to success."

- "Focus comes easy to me."

- "I am a smart, capable woman with all the skills I need to achieve this goal."

Exist loudly and proudly

What do you think of when you picture a "confident woman"? A common stereotypical image might be someone dressed to kill, speaking in public, constantly meeting new people, comfortable being the centre of attention, the life of every party — the list goes on.

It is a misconception that we should all aspire to this specific brand of confidence. Building real confidence involves:

- Accepting everything that's unique about you
- Showing up to every interaction as the most authentic version of yourself
- Being honest about who you are beneath all the layers of societal pressure
- Finding your voice and speaking up for what you believe in
- Going after the things you want out of life, regardless of fear

You are the only one of you, so don't let the world miss out on your uniqueness. Exist as loudly as you like, but exist as you. No one else can.

Stand up
for yourself

Confidence is something we can all benefit from, and one of the best things it does for us is give us the ability to stand up for ourselves. Between people-pleasing, saying sorry too much and not being able to assert our boundaries, a lack of confidence means we lack the courage needed to voice our opinion when someone or something gets in the way of our goals.

Standing up for yourself is part of protecting your boundaries, and it tells the world around you a) what your values are, and b) what you will and will not stand for. If it helps, try taking 5 minutes to make a note of your values and boundaries: for example, "I value my freedom above all else" or "I will set healthy boundaries at social events and not spend more time there than I am comfortable with." The more your confidence grows, the more comfortable you will become standing up for yourself.

Stand up for what's right

While building confidence gives us all sorts of personal gifts, others around us can also benefit from our new-found voice. It unlocks a chance to share our honest opinions on the things we truly believe in and stand up for what is right. This might mean finding the correct words to stick up for a friend who is being bullied, or it could mean lending your voice to an issue you feel strongly about.

Standing up for what's right requires you to speak up and act in the right moments, and the more your confidence develops, the more comfortable you will become with not letting injustices slip past you.

AS MY
CONFIDENCE
BUILDS, SO
DOES MY ABILITY
TO CHANGE
THE WORLD
AROUND ME

Don't wait
another second

Developing confidence can take a long time, and often, changes are so incremental that we may not even realize we are changing. Don't allow an overthinking brain to stop you from being confident for even a second longer. Some people spend years of their life listening to the voice that tells them not to speak up, not to aspire, not to try harder and not to take all the opportunities the world serves up for them.

Confidence builds the more you practise it, so try pretending that fear and shame don't exist, and don't wait another second to go after what you want. Sometimes you need to fake it till you make it!

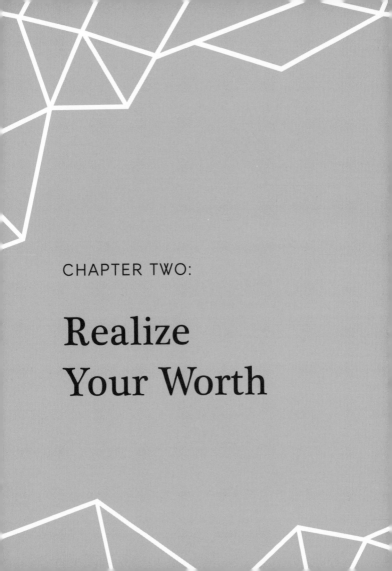

CHAPTER TWO:

Realize
Your Worth

Self-worth is like a muscle that needs to be exercised to stay strong, and after years of not using it, it may have become weakened. The tips in this chapter are designed to slowly build your self-worth again, just as you might make an exercise plan at the gym. You will learn techniques to protect yourself from external negativity and doubt, and examine the words you say to yourself internally that affect your mindset and keep you stuck. Along the way, you'll learn the power of gratitude, celebrate your strengths and begin to hype yourself up.

Building self-worth

Self-worth is the worth, or value, we see in ourselves. It can be difficult to recognize our own self-worth sometimes because often we consider it through the eyes of others. But this sense of worthiness shouldn't come from others: it's about valuing our own uniqueness and knowing that we deserve to take up space in the world.

A good way to start building your self-worth is by doing the things you enjoy and are good at. Getting good at something — and having fun while doing it — can make you feel capable and proficient. So make sure you carve out some time each day to invest in hobbies that make you feel great.

Building self-love

Self-love is the love and respect we have for ourselves. If you don't love yourself, it's harder to find the drive to speak up or protect your boundaries. Think of it this way: it's likely you would jump to your best friend's defence if the situation called for it – well, you need to be a friend to yourself, too.

The best way to cultivate self-love is by showing yourself some care and affection. Many people view self-care as bath bombs and scented candles, but true self-care is taking the time to prioritize your own needs, whatever they may be. Whether you wind down by reading a good book or going for a scenic walk, make sure you find time each day for taking care of you.

Building self-esteem

Self-esteem is our overall sense of self and how we perceive ourselves in the world. High self-esteem means we like the person we are and are confident living life as our authentic self.

To grow your self-esteem, try focusing more on your strengths and successes and forgiving yourself any mistakes (we all make them). Note down every day the things about yourself you appreciate: for example, "I'm grateful to work in a job that utilizes my skills." Taking time each day to celebrate your successes will help strengthen your relationship with the woman in the mirror.

Only make decisions
that support your self-image,
self-esteem, and self-worth.

OPRAH WINFREY

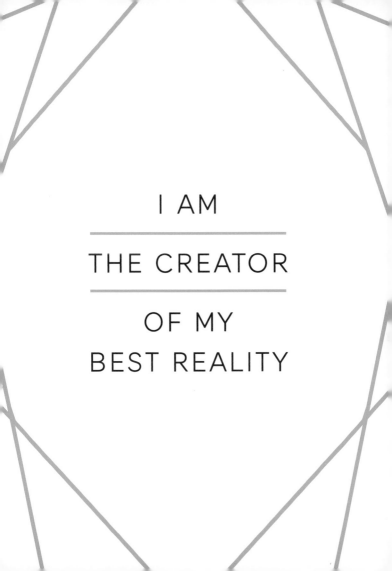

I AM

THE CREATOR

OF MY
BEST REALITY

~~Fit in~~ Stand out

Confidence and true self-worth come from the inside, and it's up to us to create them for ourselves. Instead, we often look to external sources to validate how well we fit in — whether this means dressing to impress our friends or copying what others do on social media.

It's important to remember that you are uniquely you and it's your differences that make you special. To celebrate your uniqueness, think about what you can do each day to showcase your amazing authentic self. This could mean wearing that outlandish outfit you've always shied away from or getting up to do karaoke when you're out with friends. Remember, you deserve to live unapologetically as yourself.

Attitude of gratitude

Gratitude is an underused tool that can be such a confidence booster. It is the act of appreciating the things we have in our life, and this could be as big as being grateful for our significant other or as small as being grateful for finding a good parking space.

One study found that after ten weeks, participants who wrote about gratitude regularly were more optimistic, felt better about life and exercised more than other participants.

No matter how bad your self-esteem is at the moment, you can always find something to be grateful for. Taking 5 minutes a day to note down everything you're grateful for can help to remind you of the amazing things you already have in your life.

Learn to take compliments

How many times have you been given a compliment and instantly stepped into your discomfort zone? Many of us are familiar with the feeling. You may have got used to instantly playing the compliment down; for example, when someone compliments your outfit, you say, "Thanks, it's really old." Or you might concentrate on the negatives; for example, when someone congratulates a presentation you gave, you say, "Thanks, I messed up a few times though."

A lack of confidence and self-worth can make us instantly jump to the assumption that — even if we have done something well — we are only being complimented out of politeness.

It's time to learn to take compliments like the worthy, loved, amazing woman you are. So let's turn those scenarios around. If someone compliments your outfit, say, "Thanks, I love it too." Or when they compliment your presentation skills, say, "Thanks, I'm really proud of how it went." Learning to accept compliments in a positive way, even if you don't fully believe them, will help you realize your worth over time.

Ignore the naysayers

We all come across situations and people that can easily knock our confidence and shake our self-worth. Difficult situations or challenging relationships can test how strong our self-worth really is, so we need to learn to protect it. For example, you might receive a mean comment on a picture you posted on social media or constantly be given criticism at work but no praise. All these things, over time, can start to make you feel bad about yourself.

Ignore all the negative chatter, let the naysayers do their own thing, and work on protecting your self-worth to remain positive through all of the trials life throws your way. By using the tips in this chapter daily, you'll start to feel surer of yourself, which means you'll be less inclined to take on board negative criticism.

The power of self-talk

Often, the most hurtful words come from our own minds. Self-talk is the internal thoughts we have throughout the day, which may be subconscious and barely noticeable or loud and obnoxious inside our heads, making us feel bad about ourselves.

Negative self-talk can stop us recognizing and seizing opportunities when they are in front of us, and can lead to general feelings of worthlessness. Research has even found that negative self-talk can exacerbate feelings of depression, so it's important to be mindful of what you are thinking and choose the correct course if your thoughts are taking you in the wrong direction.

Try this technique out today: if and when you find your internal monologue being self-critical, try immediately counteracting it with a positive observation instead. For example, if your brain says "I hate my smile — it's so ugly", tell yourself, "My smile is beautiful because it lights up my whole face." Adopting this as a regular habit will help you develop a more positive mindset and view of yourself.

A small step towards self-belief

Sometimes when you don't believe in yourself it can be hard to know how to take that first step towards your goals. But if you don't believe you can do something big, why not start small? For example, if you want to start your own business, why not start by attending a business seminar? Or if you want to become a stand-up comedian, why not try just writing your first joke? Take 5 minutes out of your day to think of the first step towards your goal and work on having enough self-belief to take it.

Exercise your self-belief

The wonderful thing about our self-belief is that it grows stronger the more we exercise it. Every time we prove to our brain that we can do something, it registers as a success and we add a new notch to our level of self-belief. If we do this for long enough, then one or two setbacks will do nothing to affect our level of self-belief.

Even if you feel you have zero self-belief at present, always remember this is something you can practise and improve. By affirming yourself every day (see page 31), knowing who you want to be and facing your fears, you will slowly start to feel your self-belief grow.

Address your inner critic

Do you recognize your own negative self-talk when it pops up? It's a natural function of our brain that just wants to keep us safe from fear and embarrassment by encouraging us to stay in our lane, but sometimes it needs confronting.

Try writing a letter to your inner critic and let her know why you plan to take some steps out of your comfort zone, starting now. You could start by saying, "Thank you for keeping me safe all these years" but then go on to say, "but now, I think I'm ready to face a little fear or embarrassment in order to take big steps towards my dreams." You can then expand on what you want to do and how it will help you to move towards a more confident future.

Goodbye comparison

The comparison trap is easy to fall into when we are constantly seeing what others are doing, whether that's friends, family or strangers. In our modern age, social media is a big part of why so many of us compare our own lives with others', wondering why we don't have as much, why we aren't as happy, or why we don't have the same level of confidence.

While social media can be a helpful way to keep in touch with friends and see what's going on in the world, it can have negative impacts too. To avoid this, try limiting your time spent on social media and find new things to do during prime social media hours, such as reading a book. You could also end every scrolling session by heading to your notes app to write one thing you are grateful for in your own life. Remember, being confident means celebrating your own life, not comparing it with others'.

SHE REMEMBERED
WHO SHE WAS AND
THE GAME CHANGED.

LALAH DELIA

Celebrate your wins

We are so quick to celebrate the amazing achievements of our friends, family members and colleagues, but why do we shy away from celebrating ourselves? The more you celebrate positive things that you made happen, the more your mind begins to realize you are worth celebrating.

Whether it's a big award at work, cooking from scratch, passing an exam, cleaning the oven, running one mile, having a baby, or something completely different, small or big, we should always give ourselves a pat on the back. Take some time today to reward yourself for your wins, whether that's treating yourself to your favourite snack or engaging in your most loved hobby. You deserve to be celebrated.

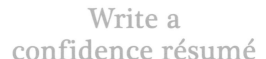

Write a confidence résumé

Résumés are usually for job applications, but what if you created one to showcase your confidence?

Take a piece of paper and list all the impressive things you've done. These don't need to be career-related, they can be things you are proud of in all areas of life, such as your home life, creative pursuits, charitable contributions, travel adventures and so on. You could divide your confidence résumé into sections, such as "experiences", "skills", "big moments" or "goals achieved". By regularly reading over your confidence résumé, you will be reminded of all the wonderful things you have to offer the world.

Promote yourself

Learning to promote yourself effectively takes time, but it is a worthwhile endeavour that can help you show up as yourself and have people take notice. A study has found that women who were more proactive in making their achievements visible tended to advance further in the workplace and experienced greater career satisfaction. With this in mind, think about the proactive steps you could take today to self-promote. Perhaps you could share your accomplishments, advocate for your contributions or provide support to your peers and colleagues.

Be your own hype woman

Imagine you are trying to boost a close friend's confidence by telling them how amazing they are and how deserving they are of an opportunity. How would you hype them up? Now, imagine the shoe is on the other foot. What do you think they would say to you? Would they question your worth, or would they give you all the motivation, love and support that you need?

Notice how easy it is for you to think kind things about your friend, compared to how difficult it is to think kind things about yourself. It's time to imagine you are your own best friend. Try writing yourself a positive pep talk to hype yourself up. Show yourself the same love, kindness and motivation that you would to others.

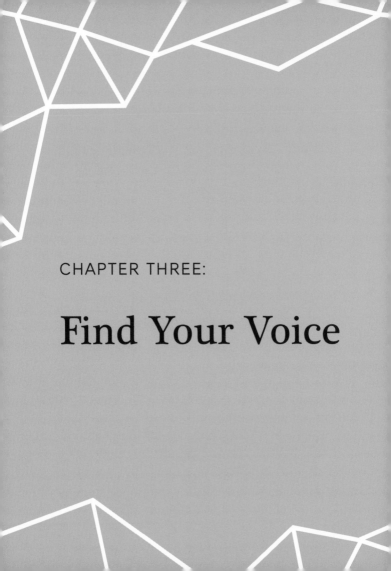

CHAPTER THREE:

Find Your Voice

When we lack confidence and self-belief for too long, the negative voice in our head takes over. As you start to develop your confidence once again, you need to listen out for your own voice.

This chapter is filled with tips and advice to help you listen closely for that quiet voice. Your inner cheerleader is still in there, you just need to turn up the volume so you can start to articulate your needs clearly, shout about your desires and speak with conviction and authority. In this way, you can build unshakeable confidence.

It took me quite a long
time to develop a voice,
and now that I have it,
I am not going to be silent.

MADELEINE K. ALBRIGHT

My voice is loud –
my voice is needed –
my voice can
change the world

Speak up

Without confidence, we might avoid speaking what is in our minds for fear of judgement. But your voice can have an incredible impact.

A great example of this is Rosa Parks, a Black woman who refused to give up her seat to a white passenger on a segregated bus in 1955. By using her voice to speak about injustice, she inadvertently played a huge part in the US civil rights movement.

Not every instance of speaking up will be quite so history-making, but it could make a difference to your life, even if in only a small way. The more you speak your mind, the more your confidence grows.

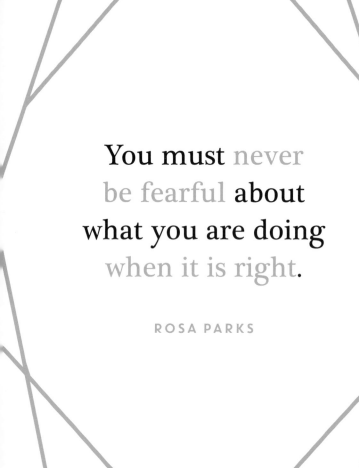

You must never
be fearful about
what you are doing
when it is right.

ROSA PARKS

How to speak up

Speaking up could mean shouting from the rooftops, but it could also mean finding the courage to speak up in a subtler way. Everyone can find their own unique way to say what's on their mind and have people listen.

Have a think about ways you could make your voice heard today. It could be something small, like asking your friend to pay you back for their share of the meal you covered, or letting the person in front of you in a queue know their bag is open. Instead of thinking "I'll just wait a little longer", get used to using your voice, in small ways at first, and feel your confidence growing.

Quit
people-pleasing

People-pleasing is the practice of avoiding conflict by saying yes to whatever someone else wants rather than speaking up about what you want. While it's harmless every so often, making it a habit can reinforce your low self-esteem, affect the honesty of your relationships and lead to resentment and unhappiness.

Make a list or mental note of some of your common people-pleasing behaviours. Think about what you could do to turn them around in a friendly way. For example, if you usually agree to working late when asked even if you're busy, try responding with something like, "I'm busy tonight, but I can help you first thing on Monday." Or if someone asks you to split a bill equally when you didn't have a starter or cocktails, politely say, "Would you mind if we each pay for what we had?" By avoiding people-pleasing and learning to advocate for yourself, you can become your own champion and have healthier relationships where your boundaries are respected.

Sorry, not sorry

The word "sorry" certainly has its place in our vocabulary, but are you guilty of apologizing too much? Many of us overuse the word "sorry"; for example, when passing someone in a tight space, asking a friend to repeat something, or feeling awkward that we made it to the printer before our colleague did.

In these examples, sorry can easily be replaced by: "Excuse me", "Could you repeat that?" or "Thanks for waiting, I'll be done soon." There is no need to make yourself feel guilty for taking up space and going about your business. Be conscious of this and see how you can avoid an unnecessary apology today.

TODAY, TOMORROW
AND EVERY DAY,
I AM CONFIDENT

Reframe your apologies

For many of us, sorry is used as an automatic reaction to awkward situations. While it isn't hurting anyone, saying sorry a lot does affect our confidence over time, as it tells our brain we have things to apologize for, and therefore feel shame for. Next time you let a sorry slip out, don't beat yourself up about it. Instead, go through these steps:

1. **Catch** – Acknowledge it silently to yourself

2. **Release** – Forgive your brain for the error

3. **Reframe** – Plan what you could say instead next time

The more you build this habit, the sooner you will be able to stop yourself before a sorry rather than after. Eventually, you will be using your replacement phrase instead.

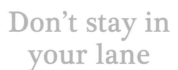

Don't stay in your lane

Trying new things is a great way to increase confidence, and you will want to do a lot of this on the road to finding your voice. Try new things, embrace new experiences, meet new people, take chances and veer from your lane regularly. Try something new today, even if only for 5 minutes. It can be something as simple as picking up a book in a genre you haven't tried before, drinking a new type of tea or taking a class to learn something new. Even if something doesn't feel very "you", try it anyway.

I AM CONFIDENT ENOUGH TO INVITE NEW AND EXCITING EXPERIENCES

Set your
boundaries

As your confidence grows, you are likely to feel more comfortable setting boundaries, which is a really helpful skill to have in all areas of life. Boundary setting doesn't have to be significant or dramatic; it can be something as simple as making it known to your friend group that you don't want to engage in gossip, or setting an out-of-office reply on your emails to let colleagues know you won't answer them after 6 p.m.

Take 5 minutes to think about your own boundaries. You might want to take into account your dislikes, stressors, the type of work you don't enjoy, what times of the day you are most and least productive and so on. Remember, never feel bad for making your boundaries clear in a kind yet direct way. Use a piece of paper to brainstorm some of your boundaries.

Take up space

Lacking confidence can feel like going through life taking up as little space as possible and trying not to get in anyone's way. Can you relate to this? While it may feel comfortable for a while, it can leave you feeling unfulfilled.

When you try to make yourself small, you are shying away from being yourself, speaking your mind, standing your ground and everything else that requires confidence. Not taking up space means not expressing yourself fully.

In finding our voice, we must learn to take up space in every room we enter and make our presence known. You are worthy of taking up space.

Command authority

Speaking up only works if you can make people listen. You don't have to speak loudly or angrily; you can speak with conviction by building a reputation as an authority on a subject or by using strong, confident body language to subconsciously encourage people to take you more seriously.

When you're trying to be authoritative, stand up straight, look people in the eye and use gestures to emphasize points. Try using clear, concise language. Ditch filler words (like "um") and spend a couple of seconds longer thinking of the correct word. You can practise this in the mirror at home to build your confidence in making your voice heard and your presence known.

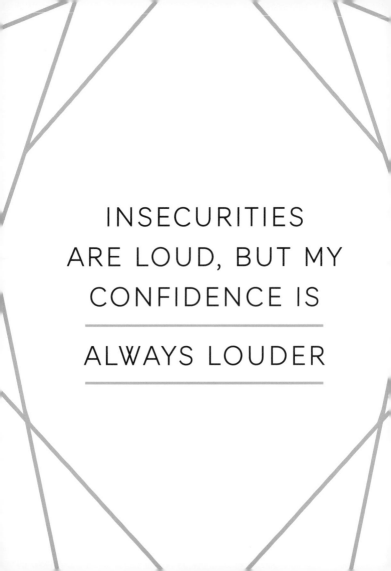

INSECURITIES
ARE LOUD, BUT MY
CONFIDENCE IS

_____

ALWAYS LOUDER

_____

Don't waste your energy trying to change opinions... Do your thing, and don't care if they like it.

TINA FEY

Meditating for confidence

Anyone – introverts and extroverts alike – can benefit from learning mindfulness techniques. These powerful tools can boost confidence by enhancing mental clarity and helping you tap into emotions. A simple internet search of guided meditations can uncover a whole host of tools for reducing stress, relaxing the nervous system, tackling self-doubt and much more. Taking the time to centre your thoughts and focus on your breath can help you tune into negative self-talk and turn it around. It can also help you calm an overthinking mind, stop ruminating, cultivate emotional resilience, observe thoughts without judgement and reframe limiting beliefs. Try practising meditation for 5 minutes every day and learn to enjoy the present moment.

YOU HAVE
BEEN CRITICIZING
YOURSELF FOR YEARS,
AND IT HASN'T WORKED.
TRY APPROVING
YOURSELF AND SEE
WHAT HAPPENS.

LOUISE HAY

Breathe your way to confidence

Another great mindful tool to use for times when you need to boost your confidence is breathwork. While this won't necessarily make you confident right away, it can help you relax, slow a racing heart and steady your mind ahead of a stressful situation.

Breathwork gives you a calm space to prepare for pushing those comfort zone boundaries so you can approach challenges with a confident mindset. So if you need a quick confidence boost, try the 4-7-8 method, which involves breathing in for four counts, holding your breath for seven and then exhaling for eight. This tool can be used to calm anxiety, which can sometimes mask feelings of confidence.

Confidence
for introverts

Many people mistake introversion for being shy, but it is possible to be a confident introvert. This simply means you might need to change your perception of what confidence really means. It could be feeling confident enough to say no to plans you don't want to join in on so you can recharge your batteries for another social event. Or it could be having a handful of very close friends rather than aspiring to have a large group of acquaintances.

If you identify as an introvert, it's time to fully embrace this part of your personality and stop apologizing for it. Remind yourself every day that, as an introvert, you are still worthy of speaking your mind and sharing your ideas with the world.

The "3, 2, 1, Go!" technique

When it comes to taking action on things we want to do, we can end up overthinking them so much that we lose the moment and retreat back into our shell. There will always be a reason not to take action, but when you are faced with the choice, you can use the 3, 2, 1, Go! method to interrupt rumination before it has a chance to take hold.

It's as simple as it sounds. The second your brain starts to feed you reasons why you shouldn't do something, think to yourself "3, 2, 1, Go!" and act immediately by taking the first step. This approach allows you to make a gut and heart decision rather than applying the logic which leads to overthinking. It isn't always wise to jump in without thinking, but trust that you will know the right situations to use this tool when they arise.

The superwoman stance

The superwoman stance was discovered as a result of research done by social psychologist Amy Cuddy and is thought to improve confidence ahead of stressful moments. All you need to do is stand up tall, place your feet a little wider than hip-width apart, pull your shoulders back and lift your chin up.

Research suggests that by standing like superwoman, you can project confidence to others and essentially "cheat" your brain into believing you are confident. The stance is thought to increase your overall sense of self-worth, and the research even found that power posing for 2 minutes lowered the stress hormone cortisol in study participants. So try adopting this powerful stance today.

I don't focus on
what I'm up against.
I focus on my goals and
I try to ignore the rest.

VENUS WILLIAMS

CHAPTER FOUR:

Follow
Your Dreams

When we lack self-love, we also lack an inner belief in ourselves. Not only does this mean we feel incapable of achieving a goal, we may also feel unworthy of achieving it. If you want to follow your dreams, the first step is to develop an unshakeable self-belief that will carry you through the difficult moments ahead – and yes, all dream-chasing requires some level of discomfort and difficulty.

Whatever your ambition in life – from the tiny bucket list item to the enormous goal that could change your life forever – this chapter can assist you in finding the confidence you need to pursue it.

I am slowly
creating the
kind of life I
dream about

Your short-term bucket list

A bucket list is typically thought of as a list of things you would like to do in your whole life, but that can be a little overwhelming to think about! Instead, why not make a bucket list for a shorter period of time?

Use a piece of paper to brainstorm what you would like to do in the next three months, six months, year, three years, five years, ten years or whatever time period you'd like to set yourself. The choice is up to you. Don't worry about the level of confidence you think you will need in order to achieve something, just write it down and tackle it when you feel ready.

Believe you can and you're halfway there.

THEODORE ROOSEVELT

Excuses, excuses

Any time our confidence is in question, excuses seem to pop up like whack-a-moles. These self-imposed mental blocks will hold us back as we progress towards our goals.

Sometimes excuses are valid and required in order to impose our personal boundaries, but they can often be an automatic reaction to the thought of moving out of our comfort zone, and making them too frequently becomes a habit that limits our long-term potential.

When you find yourself coming up with excuses to avoid going after your dreams, try counteracting them with some kind advice, just like you would with a friend. For example, if you tell yourself you're not skilled enough so why bother chasing your goals, tell yourself: "You have all the skills to achieve everything you want."

"I could never"

Have you ever used the phrase "I could *never* do that"? If you find yourself thinking this, put your thoughts under scrutiny: could I really *never* do this?

If you think of something scary that you find near impossible to carry out in reality, break down the steps to show exactly how you would — and could — do it. For example, if you believe you could never have the courage to ask your boss for a raise, plan some steps towards achieving this, such as researching what others in your role are paid, making a folder of data on the value you have added to the company then booking a meeting with your boss and so on. Being able to practically and realistically visualize the path to success will help you banish "I could never" for good.

Your
comfort zone

The comfort zone is a lovely place. It's decorated with all your favourite colours and patterns. The lighting is just right. It's cosy, warm and totally safe. No one else can get into your comfort zone, so you are free to be however you want to be in there.

The problem is that everything exciting and amazing that is worth pursuing in life lies outside the boundaries of the comfort zone. While it may be desirable to stay safe and warm inside the impenetrable comfort zone, real confidence is built when you push those boundaries until your comfort zone expands and you feel comfortable doing more and more things.

Carve out 5 minutes each day to try something outside of your comfort zone. Start with something small, such as trying a new food, and then build towards bigger steps over time. By gradually moving out of your comfort zone, you'll be amazed to see just how much you are capable of.

Worst-case scenarios

When doing something outside of your comfort zone, a great question to consider is: what's the worst that can happen? In many cases, you will notice that the absolute worst-case scenario really isn't that bad and is something you can plan for. Think about what the worst-case scenario is in pursuing your goal. What makes you feel uncomfortable and unconfident? These are the things that lie outside of your comfort zone, and they are worth chasing after.

Try using "what's the worst that can happen?" as a journalling prompt. Writing this out will help you see what you're up against and make you realize that these obstacles are not as intimidating as they might at first seem.

The discomfort list

If you can get comfortable with being uncomfortable, you can achieve pretty much anything you set your mind to. Discomfort is the feeling that holds us back, and learning to lean into this feeling can be helpful for figuring out where our confidence drops off.

Make a list of the things that make you uncomfortable. This could be something like being unprepared for exams, getting your picture taken, meeting new people and so on.

Try to find a common thread between some of the things you list. Is there a theme emerging? If you learned to ignore your inner critic and carry on with these uncomfortable situations regardless, what might you be able to achieve?

Build your skills

One research project found that, despite performing equally well on a science quiz, female participants underestimated their performance due to having a lower opinion of their scientific reasoning skills.

A sure-fire way to improve your confidence in almost any area is to up-level your skills. The more we learn about certain subjects, the more we feel we can confidently discuss them with others without feelings of imposter syndrome taking over.

Think about skills you might want to build. These could be to help with your professional development, to explore something you have always been curious about, to hone your creative practice, or something else. Try to make time every day to work on and build these skills, and you'll be one step closer to achieving your goals.

The bounce-back checklist

Setbacks will happen as you move towards the more confident version of yourself, but the great thing is, bouncing back from them becomes easier and easier as you build your self-esteem.

Creating a bounce-back checklist could help streamline the process of getting back on track. This is a list of steps you can take to bounce back from failures, and it can be helpful to refer to when your mind is busy focusing on the negatives. If you can't think of positives after a setback, just look at your list and get started.

An example list might include things like journalling on how the setback makes you feel, reaching out to a friend to share those feelings, meditating for 5 minutes until any feelings of embarrassment start to ease and so on. Create your own bounce-back checklist and refer to it whenever you face challenges or setbacks.

Affirmations for bouncing back

Affirmations can be useful in times when we need some words of encouragement to pick ourselves back up off the floor.

Here are a few affirmations that could help you to bounce back after a setback:

- "I am grateful for the lessons this setback can teach me."
- "Every successful person in the world has experienced setbacks, so I'm in good company."
- "Setbacks don't affect me. My confidence is a shield."
- "When you are as passionate about the goal as I am, bouncing back is easy."
- "I will never stop trying to reach my goals."

Discover
your passions

What makes you curious about the world? Finding your passions and making time each day for them can be a great way to boost your day-to-day confidence as well as your happiness. Identify the things that make you want to learn more, do more, create more and so on.

A great way to approach this is to imagine you are a level ten confident woman and have the potential to do anything. Anything at all. Where would you start? Find what makes you curious and start there.

One excellent question to help with this is: what would you try if you knew you couldn't fail?

WHY SHOULD I CARE
WHAT OTHER PEOPLE
THINK OF ME?
I AM WHO I AM.
AND WHO I WANNA BE.

AVRIL LAVIGNE

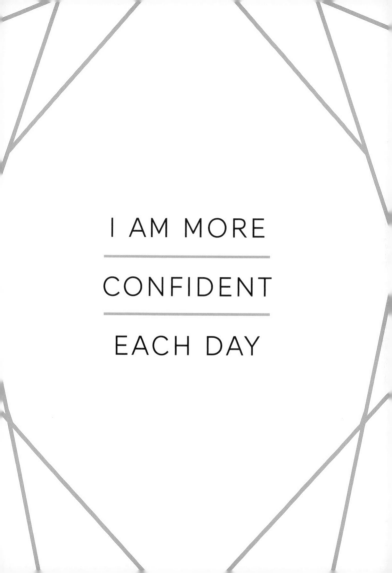

I AM MORE

CONFIDENT

EACH DAY

Don't seek permission

A great confidence hack that's easy to implement in our daily life is to stop asking for permission for everything we do. Checking in before we make decisions to ensure we are making the right one can be an automatic reaction, even though we should have enough self-belief to make the decision confidently ourselves.

Delayed actions lead to missed opportunities, but learning to jump in and make fast decisions based on our own experience and knowledge can be the difference between getting something we have always wanted and letting it slip through our fingers.

OUTSIDE OF MY
COMFORT ZONE
IS WHERE THE
ADVENTURE STARTS
HAPPENING

Do one thing
every day that
scares you.

ELEANOR ROOSEVELT

Drive towards your goals

Goals give us something to strive for and a direction to travel in. Whether you already have goals in mind or you are exploring which ones you would like to work on, this chapter is like your goal roadmap encouraging you to set ambitious targets and start driving towards them with your new-found confidence in the passenger seat.

If you haven't yet decided what those goals are, that's OK. Start to consider what these might be based on the values you have discovered in earlier chapters.

Fiercely protect your goals

How many times have you said the phrases "I always wanted to..." or "Someday I will..."? If you have a graveyard of great ideas, abandoned creative pursuits and "somedays" in your mind, it is never, ever too late to take action.

Whether your life plans were derailed in some way, you feel the confidence gap has a lot to answer for or you have simply never been able to prioritize the things you want in life, make today the day you start to fiercely protect the goals that matter to you.

Set mini goals

Research shows that sticking to incremental achievements (or mini goals) can help to boost your motivation early on in the journey to your larger goals.

Try writing down your goals and breaking them into smaller, bite-sized steps. For example, if your goal is to run a marathon but this feels out of your reach right now, create mini goals you can tick off each day so that you feel a constant sense of achievement. These could include "buy new trainers", "map out a route", "find a training plan online", "run my first kilometre" and so on. Not only does this make your bigger goal seem much less daunting, it also makes it much more achievable.

Schedule your goals

You know what your goals are. You know when you're most confident. Now it's time to prioritize your goals by making sure they appear before anything else in your weekly planner or monthly calendar.

Many of us start with things like work, appointments, social events and so on, and we are eventually left with no room in the week for the things that are arguably most important to us. Making sure that working on your goals has a space in your calendar is the best way to prioritize it above all else. So quit procrastinating and pencil it in!

Loving yourself isn't vanity. It's sanity.

KATRINA MAYER

Conclusion

Developing confidence is a lifetime pursuit, but this book contains the actionable advice you need to take big steps towards a more confident version of yourself. You can revisit the tips within these pages whenever you are feeling shy or lacking belief in yourself, or if you just want an extra dose of confidence ahead of a big moment.

It won't always feel like an easy journey, but the more you practise building your confidence, the better you will start to feel about yourself and the easier it will be to move towards your goals.

No matter what level of confidence you feel you currently have, there are lots of ways you can improve it and start to show up as a bolder, brighter version of yourself with plenty of self-belief to boot. So keep these pearls of wisdom in mind wherever you go, and start showing up as the most confident version of yourself every day.

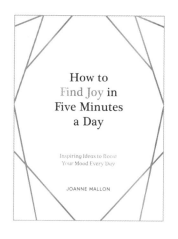

HOW TO FIND JOY IN FIVE MINUTES A DAY

Inspiring Ideas to Boost Your Mood Every Day

Joanne Mallon

Hardback

ISBN: 978-1-80007-156-8

Joy is everywhere once you know where to look

This beautiful book includes tips and ideas to help you elevate your mood and liven up your routine. Perhaps you will try setting an intention, performing a small act of kindness, or eating outdoors in the fresh air. Even the smallest moment of positivity can transform your outlook, so whether you follow one tip or many, you are sure to lift your spirits and find a small oasis of happiness every day – all you need is five minutes.

HOW TO FIND CALM IN FIVE MINUTES A DAY

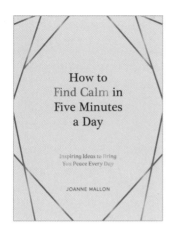

Inspiring Ideas to Bring You Peace Every Day

Joanne Mallon

Hardback

ISBN: 978-1-83799-010-8

Calm is everywhere once you know where to look

This beautiful book includes tips and ideas to help you recentre yourself and rise above everyday stresses. Perhaps you will try incorporating mindfulness into your routine, visualizing what calm looks like to you, or writing down your worries. Even the smallest moment of calm can transform your outlook, so whether you follow one tip or many, you're sure to find clarity and calm every day – all you need is five minutes.

Have you enjoyed this book?

If so, why not write a review
on your favourite website?

If you're interested in finding out
more about our books, find us on
Facebook at Summersdale Publishers,
on Twitter/X at @Summersdale
and on Instagram and TikTok at
@summersdalebooks and get in
touch. We'd love to hear from you!

Thanks very much for buying
this Summersdale book.

www.summersdale.com